issues today

HIV and AIDS

KV-191-977

Contents

…pendence.co.uk

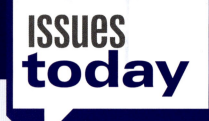

A resource for KS3

About Key Stage 3

Key Stage 3 refers to the first three years of secondary schooling, normally years 7, 8 and 9, during which pupils are aged between 11 and 14.

This series is also suitable for Scottish P7, S1 and S2 students.

About Issues Today

Issues Today is a series of resource books on contemporary social issues for Key Stage 3 pupils. It is based on the concept behind the popular *Issues* series for 14- to 18-year-olds, also published by Independence.

Each volume contains information from a variety of sources, including government reports and statistics, newspaper and magazine articles, surveys and polls, academic research and literature from charities and lobby groups. The information has been tailored to an 11 to 14 age group; it has been rewritten and presented in a simple, straightforward format to be accessible to Key Stage 3 pupils.

In addition, each *Issues Today* title features handy tasks and assignments based on the information contained in the book, for use in class, for homework or as a revision aid.

Issues Today can be used as a learning resource in a variety of Key Stage 3 subjects, including English, Science, History, Geography, PSHE, Citizenship, Sex and Relationships Education and Religious Education.

About this book

HIV and AIDS is the twenty-eighth volume in the *Issues Today* series. It looks at the AIDS epidemic in the developing world and at issues surrounding HIV and AIDS in the UK. It also looks at current treatments and strategies to tackle the growing epidemic.

HIV and AIDS offers a useful overview of the many issues involved in this topic. However, at the end of each article is a URL for the relevant organisation's website, which can be visited by pupils who want to carry out further research.

Because the information in this book is gathered from a number of different sources, pupils should think about the origin of the text and critically evaluate the information that is presented. Does the source have a particular bias or agenda? Are you being presented with facts or opinions? Do you agree with the writer?

At the end of each chapter there are two pages of activities relating to the articles and issues raised in that chapter. The 'Brainstorm' questions can be done as a group or individually after reading the articles. This should prompt some ideas and lead on to further activities. Some suggestions for such activities are given under the headings 'Oral', 'Moral Dilemmas', 'Research', 'Written' and 'Design' that follow the 'Brainstorm' questions.

For more information about *Issues Today* and its sister series, *Issues* (for pupils aged 14 to 18), please visit the Independence website.

www.independence.co.uk

HIV and AIDS

HUMAN IMMUNODEFICIENCY VIRUS (HIV) is an infection. It's passed from person to person by having sex without using a condom, using needles with infected blood on them, having a blood transfusion or organ donation from someone with the virus, and from mother to baby.

AIDS (Acquired Immune Deficiency Syndrome) happens when the immune system has been weakened so much by HIV that it can't fight certain life-threatening infections and illnesses.

Worldwide, it is estimated that over 40 million people are living with HIV and around three million people die each year from AIDS-related illnesses.

HIV and the immune system

The immune system protects your body against infection. An important part of the system is white blood cells. These cells find and kill invading germs, such as bacteria and viruses, stopping serious diseases developing and damaging your body. HIV is able to avoid being destroyed by the immune system by regularly changing its outer 'coat'. It multiplies (replicates) inside the special type of white blood cells called CD4 cells. These cells normally help other types of immune cell to attack and kill disease-causing germs.

As HIV multiplies, it destroys CD4 cells, so there are less of them. This means that the body's ability to fight infection is weakened.

HIV in the UK

The number of people living with HIV in the UK has gone up steadily since the 1980s when the virus was discovered. Official figures for 2005 put this at nearly 63,500 people.

Most HIV infections in the UK occur in gay men. Passing on the virus heterosexually has gone up a lot in recent years. However, most of these infections are in people who have come to live in the UK from countries where HIV is common and have been diagnosed since living in the UK.

> **Worldwide, it is estimated that over 40 million people are living with HIV and around three million people die each year from AIDS-related illnesses.**

Causes

HIV can only be passed to someone else when there is enough of the virus in the blood or other body fluids to be passed to another person.

HIV infection can be passed through blood, semen, breast milk and vaginal fluids. This means HIV can be passed on during unprotected sex.

The virus can be passed from mother to baby if she has

HIV during pregnancy, childbirth or when breastfeeding. HIV can also be passed on if infected needles are used for injections, piercings or tattoos.

HIV is not found in high enough levels in other body fluids such as saliva, sweat, urine or on the skin to cause an infection from contact with these fluids.

HIV can't be passed on through normal day-to-day activities, such as sharing cutlery, sitting on toilet seats or by shaking hands.

HIV and AIDS

HIV and blood or organ donation

In the past, people have been infected with HIV through blood or organ donations. All donations in the UK are now checked for HIV, so the chances of this happening are very low.

DID YOU KNOW? *The immune system protects the body from getting serious illnesses. The HIV virus weakens the immune system so that eventually it can no longer fight diseases – this is called having AIDS. People with AIDS can die of illnesses which the immune system might normally be able to fight off, such as pneumonia.*

Symptoms

The time straight after a person becomes infected with HIV is called primary HIV infection. At this point they are very infectious because the level of the virus is high in the blood. They will have symptoms of HIV infection but may miss them because they are like other infections such as flu. Early symptoms usually start about two to six weeks after first getting HIV and last about five to ten days. Some symptoms may last longer.

After the early symptoms, HIV may not be noticed for a number of years until a person's ability to fight infections is reduced. When this happens the number of cells which fight infections has gone down so much that the body's immune system can't work properly. If a person gets certain life-threatening illnesses it is known as AIDS or advanced HIV disease.

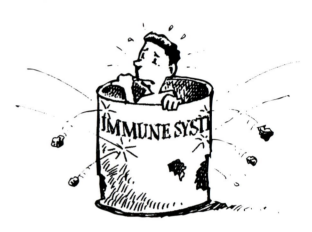

AIDS

Once the immune system has been damaged, infections appear. Common infections include a type of pneumonia called pneumocystis, and tuberculosis.

Other AIDS-related illnesses can include:

▶ various cancers;
▶ fungal, bacterial or viral infections;
▶ sight problems;
▶ dementia.

66 *There is no cure for HIV, but treatment with anti-HIV medicines slows down the progress of the disease and has reduced the number of deaths caused by AIDS-related illnesses.* **99**

Signs of primary HIV include:

▶ fever;
▶ swollen glands;
▶ sore throat;
▶ rash on the body or face;
▶ painful muscles or joints;
▶ headache;
▶ feeling sick and vomiting;
▶ ulcers on the mouth, genitals and oesophagus (tube that goes to the stomach).

HIV and AIDS

Treatment

There is no cure for HIV, but treatment with anti-HIV medicines slows down the progress of the disease and has reduced the number of deaths caused by AIDS-related illnesses. When taken properly, anti-HIV medicines mean a person with HIV could live nearly as long as someone who doesn't have the infection.

> **In the past, people have been infected with HIV through blood or organ donations. All donations in the UK are now checked for HIV, so the chances of this happening are very low.**

People known to be HIV-positive are checked regularly by doctors. Usually, once the number of CD4 white blood cells has fallen to a low level, a specialist will recommend starting drug treatment.

Medication

Anti-HIV medicines stop the virus from multiplying in the body. This lowers the amount of virus in the blood and allows the immune system to recover. To achieve this, three antiretroviral medicines are usually taken together. This combination therapy is called Highly Active Antiretroviral Therapy (HAART) and has cut the number of deaths from AIDS-related illnesses a lot.

January 2008

DID YOU KNOW?
Although there are medicines which can slow down how quickly the HIV virus damages the immune system, there is no medicine which can cure HIV or AIDS.

www.bupa.co.uk

The above information is reprinted with kind permission from Bupa.
© Bupa

Living with HIV

In countries where it is hard to get HIV treatment, AIDS-related illness is a common cause of death. In the UK, most people with HIV can get anti-HIV medicines and go on to lead full and active lives.

HIV and AIDS in the UK

Reported HIV and AIDS cases in the UK, 1990-2006.

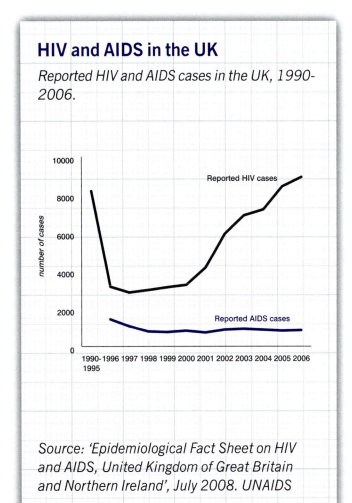

Source: 'Epidemiological Fact Sheet on HIV and AIDS, United Kingdom of Great Britain and Northern Ireland', July 2008. UNAIDS

Mini glossary

transfusion – to transfer blood from one body to another

immune system – used by the body to fight off disease

heterosexually – relating to sexual attraction between people of opposite sexes

diagnosed – when a doctor has identified that someone has a certain illness

HIV in developing countries

If there's so much AIDS in developing countries, everyone over there must know about it. So why is it still spreading?

Millions of people around the world can't get good healthcare information in their area and often do not hear about HIV and AIDS until it is too late. Also, knowing information is only a small part of changing behaviour (ask any smoker you know!). To understand the spread of the virus, we need to understand what life is like in poor countries.

> **Millions of people around the world can't get good healthcare information in their area and often do not hear about HIV and AIDS until it is too late. 99**

All these countries are so far away – AIDS over there doesn't affect me.

AIDS is having such a terrible effect on the working people of so many countries that the effects are being felt by companies and consumers all over the world. Lost people mean lost markets and lost profit. But more importantly, morally our final aim should be lives free from unnecessary suffering. HIV and AIDS is a condition which can be prevented and managed. We all have a responsibility to save suffering and lives, and our governments – who answer directly to the people – play a huge part in helping to make this happen.

When will people stop having unsafe sex? Doesn't everyone know how to use a condom now?

'After I became ill and tested HIV-positive I discovered that both my husband and his family knew that he had HIV before we were married.' This woman from Kousalya, India, is not alone in her experience.

Preventing HIV is more difficult than just telling people to use condoms. For example, in many parts of the world having a lot of children is a way for couples to become more important in their community. Everyone has the right to choose whether to have children or not – and everyone knows it is not possible to have children while using condoms.

It is also estimated that even in the United States, where access to information, HIV testing and treatment is good, 25% of people with HIV do not know they are HIV-positive. This number is a lot higher in developing countries.

> **After I became ill and tested HIV positive I discovered that both my husband and his family knew that he had HIV before we were married. 99**

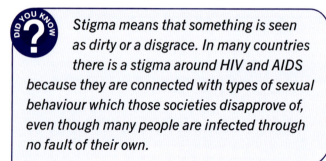

DID YOU KNOW? *Stigma means that something is seen as dirty or a disgrace. In many countries there is a stigma around HIV and AIDS because they are connected with types of sexual behaviour which those societies disapprove of, even though many people are infected through no fault of their own.*

HIV in developing countries

How can there be stigma around HIV and AIDS in developing countries when so many people have the illness?

We all know that stigma surrounds HIV and AIDS, but there is a common belief that there is less stigma about HIV and AIDS in developing countries because so many people are affected. This is not true. Societies everywhere are built on certain morals and ideas about acceptable behaviour – often relating to sex. In many African countries, for instance, women whose husbands have died of AIDS are sent away from their homes and communities because, even though it is considered okay for men to have several wives and sexual partners, the wives are almost always blamed for their husbands' HIV infection. Prejudice and fear are common and without help such as government welfare support and women's shelters, women and children in particular (often HIV-positive themselves) find they are left with no money, home or belongings and without the skills to find work.

Anyone living with HIV in a developing country will tell you that the stigma applies everywhere, and people often hide having HIV for safety reasons. All over the world the association of HIV with sexual behaviour, illness and death and particularly with stigmatised issues such as homosexuality and drug use means that fighting HIV is more difficult. ActionAid works to challenge the stigma and prejudice that surround HIV and AIDS.

Why is HIV such a problem in poor countries?

Poverty is one of the biggest causes of the spread of HIV, and of HIV-positive people getting worse until they have AIDS. Fighting HIV and AIDS in societies where the most important thing for most people is finding enough food for the family each day will always be difficult.

Poor people in developing countries are often faced with difficult choices such as going hungry that night, or making money in whatever way possible to put food on the table. Often this involves selling sex, which puts them at more risk of HIV.

While the first choice involves immediate and definite risks (hunger), the second involves only possible risk (HIV infection). Even in countries where HIV rates are as high as 39%, there is still a 61% chance of not becoming infected. And even if a person does become infected, it is often some years before illness sets in. It is a risk some have no choice but to take.

If so many people in developing countries have HIV and AIDS they must be used to dealing with it by now, and anyway, if AIDS doesn't get them something else will.

People should never have to get used to dealing with pain, tragedy and illness. HIV and AIDS break down communities and lives and although those affected do find ways of coping, there is so much that could be done internationally. Everybody has the right to a healthy life, and it is the responsibility of us all to help others around the world to achieve this.

The above information is reprinted with kind permission from ActionAid.
© ActionAid

Mini glossary

developing countries – *countries which are less developed than those in the west, meaning their citizens usually have a lower standard of living*

prejudice – *a dislike of someone or something which is based on stereotypes rather than facts*

www.actionaid.org.uk

Record UK HIV diagnoses

THE LATEST STATISTICS FROM THE HEALTH PROTECTION AGENCY show that the number of people living with HIV in the UK went up to an estimated 77,400 in 2007, with 7,734 new diagnoses in 2007 alone. Although high, the number of people diagnosed with HIV each year seems to have become stable – but this hides more worrying trends.

Increase in HIV being passed on heterosexually in the UK

The estimated number of HIV-positive people diagnosed who were infected through heterosexual contact in the UK has increased from 540 new diagnoses in 2003 to 960 in 2007, and has doubled from 11 per cent to 23 per cent as a percentage of all heterosexual diagnoses during this time.

> **Almost one in five people with diagnosed HIV who are at the point when a doctor would recommend starting treatment have made the decision not to start treatment.**

DID YOU KNOW? *HIV-positive people who take the antiretroviral medicines which can suppress the virus have a much higher life expectancy than those who don't.*

Deborah Jack, Chief Executive of NAT (National AIDS Trust), says:

> Each year a significant number of people are diagnosed with HIV, showing we still have much more to do to reduce ongoing HIV infection in the UK. Funding for prevention and testing must be increased and the Government must begin to take seriously the public health challenge of HIV in the UK, as it is growing each year.

Most worrying is the number of people who should be on HIV treatment but who in fact are not – whether because they are unaware of their infection or because they are opting not to start treatment when recommended. Treatment for HIV has revolutionised the condition and people with HIV can now expect a good life expectancy if they are diagnosed early and take their medication as advised. By not getting treatment, people are risking their healths.

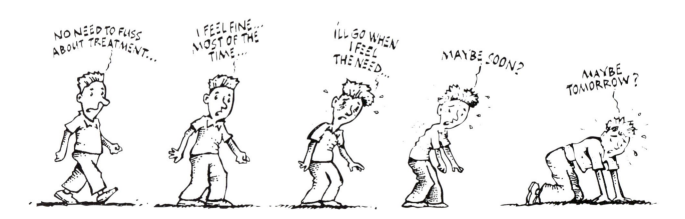

NO NEED TO FUSS ABOUT TREATMENT...

I FEEL FINE... MOST OF THE TIME...

ILL GO WHEN I FEEL THE NEED...

MAYBE SOON?

MAYBE TOMORROW?

Record UK HIV diagnoses

Many people risking health by delaying treatment

The statistics also show something else to be concerned about – the number of people choosing not to start or to delay starting treatment. Almost one in five people with diagnosed HIV who are at the point when a doctor would recommend starting treatment have made the decision not to do so.

Need to get better at diagnosing HIV early

Over a quarter (28 per cent) of people living with HIV don't know they have the infection and many of those that are diagnosed are being diagnosed late – after the point at which they should have started treatment. 42 per cent of heterosexual men and 36 per cent of heterosexual women were diagnosed late compared to 19 per cent of gay or bisexual men. People diagnosed late are 13 times more likely to die within a year of diagnosis.

> ❝ *Each year a significant number of people are diagnosed with HIV, showing we still have much more to do to reduce ongoing HIV infection in the UK.* ❞

1 December 2008

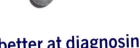

www.worldaidsday.org

The above information is reprinted with kind permission from the National AIDS Trust. © National AIDS Trust

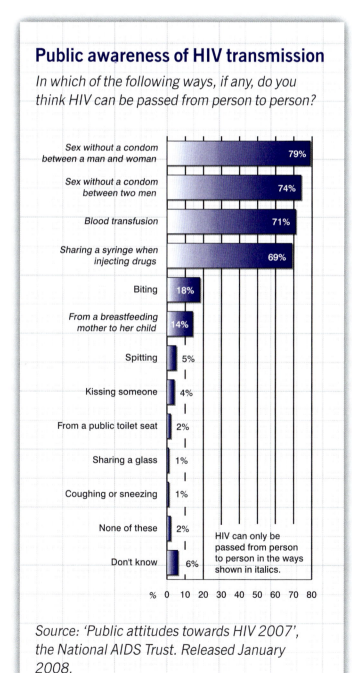

Public awareness of HIV transmission

In which of the following ways, if any, do you think HIV can be passed from person to person?

Way	%
Sex without a condom between a man and woman	79%
Sex without a condom between two men	74%
Blood transfusion	71%
Sharing a syringe when injecting drugs	69%
Biting	18%
From a breastfeeding mother to her child	14%
Spitting	5%
Kissing someone	4%
From a public toilet seat	2%
Sharing a glass	1%
Coughing or sneezing	1%
None of these	2%
Don't know	6%

HIV can only be passed from person to person in the ways shown in italics.

% 0 10 20 30 40 50 60 70 80

Source: 'Public attitudes towards HIV 2007', the National AIDS Trust. Released January 2008.

Mini glossary

bisexual – *someone who will form relationships with people of the opposite or same sex*

significant – *important*

opting – *choosing*

revolutionised – *changed drastically (for the better)*

What do you know about AIDS?

1 HIV/AIDS is a disease which mainly affects gay people.

☐ true ☐ false

2 HIV/AIDS is a fatal disease.

☐ true ☐ false

3 You can catch HIV/AIDS by sharing a drinking glass with an infected person.

☐ true ☐ false

4 Mothers can pass HIV/AIDS on to their babies during pregnancy, birth and breastfeeding.

☐ true ☐ false

5 Having sex with someone infected with HIV/AIDS is the only way you can get HIV/AIDS.

☐ true ☐ false

6 HIV/AIDS is only a problem in the developing world.

☐ true ☐ false

7 Using a condom reduces the chances of you becoming infected with HIV/AIDS.

☐ true ☐ false

8 HIV/AIDS can now be cured.

☐ true ☐ false

Public attitudes to HIV

Following are a number of statements about HIV and AIDS. Could you please indicate how strongly you agree or disagree with each of them?

Statement	Strongly agree	Tend to agree	Neither/nor	Tend to disagree	Strongly disagree	Don't know
There is still a great deal of stigma in the UK today around HIV and AIDS	26%	43%	14%	7%		8%
People who become infected with HIV through unprotected sex only have themselves to blame	18%	29%	21%	18%	8%	6
People who become infected with HIV through using drugs only have themselves to blame	31%	34%	15%	11%	4	5
More needs to be done to tackle prejudice against people living with HIV in the UK	29%	42%	16%	5		7
HIV is no longer a serious issue in the UK	3	6	10	30%	43%	8%
I think the government is doing enough to tackle HIV in the UK	3	16%	24%	29%	16%	13%

Source: 'Public attitudes towards HIV 2007', the National AIDS Trust. Released January 2008.

What do you know about AIDS?

Answers

1. HIV/AIDS is a disease which mainly affects gay people.

False. AIDS was first discovered among gay people in the USA but around the world it affects anyone and everyone. More people have been infected with HIV/AIDS through heterosexual sex than in any other way.

3. You can catch HIV/AIDS by sharing a drinking glass with an infected person.

False. The human immunodeficiency virus (HIV) cannot live for very long outside the human body. You cannot catch HIV/AIDS by sharing drinking glasses, using the same toilets or touching a person infected with HIV/AIDS.

5. Having sex with someone infected with HIV/AIDS is the only way you can get HIV/AIDS.

False. Drug users who share needles, people who are given blood transfusions or blood products in countries where the blood has not been checked for HIV and babies born to HIV-positive women can all be infected with HIV/AIDS.

7. Using a condom reduces the chances of you becoming infected with HIV/AIDS.

True. Safe sex using a condom is one of the most effective ways of stopping the spread of HIV/AIDS between sexual partners.

2. HIV/AIDS is a fatal disease.

True. HIV/AIDS weakens the body's immune system. Eventually anyone infected with HIV will die of AIDS itself or of the other diseases which they get because of their damaged immune system.

4. Mothers can pass HIV/AIDS on to their babies during pregnancy, birth and breastfeeding.

True. Women who have HIV/AIDS can pass the virus on to their children before or during birth. Even if the baby is born healthy, it may be infected during the time it is being breastfed, as the virus is found in the mother's milk.

6. HIV/AIDS is only a problem in the developing world.

False. Although the great majority of people infected with HIV/AIDS live in the developing world, HIV/AIDS is a problem everywhere, including the UK – about 700-900 people die of HIV/AIDS each year in the UK alone.

8. HIV/AIDS can now be cured.

False. Although treatments are much better than they were, and there are drugs which can delay full-blown AIDS for many years, there are still no drugs which can cure HIV/AIDS or vaccines which can protect people against it.

The stigma of HIV and AIDS

RESEARCH PUBLISHED ON 26 November 2007 shows that one in seven young people interviewed in Britain would not be willing to stay friends with someone if they had HIV and only 32% are worried about getting HIV.

The Ipsos MORI/British Red Cross survey shows that there is a worrying level of complacency and stigma towards HIV in Britain today, even though a report from UNAIDS has found that it is increasing in the UK.

Alyson Lewis, HIV Advisor at the British Red Cross, said:

66 The stigma and secrecy attached to HIV is having a direct impact on young people's ability worldwide to access information and talk openly about their fears and concerns about the spread of this devastating pandemic.

Almost half of British young people interviewed would want to keep it a secret if a member of their family was living with HIV. Many young people view HIV as a shameful secret, and we need to ensure that we demystify these fears and help young people to be more aware of the risks and how to protect themselves. 99

Nicola Waghorn (22), a Red Cross peer educator from Brighton, said:

66 I don't think young people in the UK really know that much about HIV. Many of them don't know enough about the risks involved. I can help my friends understand more by passing on information that I know and correcting their misunderstandings. 99

Hamza (20), Red Cross peer educator in Ethiopia, said:

66 I know what HIV is doing to my society. I think that if I teach one person about HIV then they can go back and teach their family. In this way awareness will come. 99

The level of stigma in Britain is similar to results from South Africa, where almost a fifth of young people interviewed would not be willing to remain friends with someone with HIV. With more than five million people living with HIV, South Africa is the country with the largest number of HIV infections in the world. In Kyrgyzstan, where HIV is starting to be noticed as a serious health problem, almost half of young people interviewed said they would not remain friends with a person living with HIV. In Ethiopia, almost a quarter (23%) of those interviewed would not be willing to remain friends with someone with HIV.

The British Red Cross supports peer education programmes at home and abroad, which enable young people to gain and share information and skills. There are thousands of young peer educators who volunteer for the Red Cross who want to help reduce stigma and discrimination towards HIV.

Lewis added: 'Our priority is to reduce stigma and promote human dignity for all people living with HIV. This campaign succeeds in that it enables young people from all over the world to talk about their experiences in their own words.'

26 November 2007

The stigma of HIV and AIDS

Awareness and understanding of HIV and AIDS

Selected findings from the British Red Cross/Ipsos MORI survey.

Which, if any, of the following would you be willing to do? Please select all that apply.

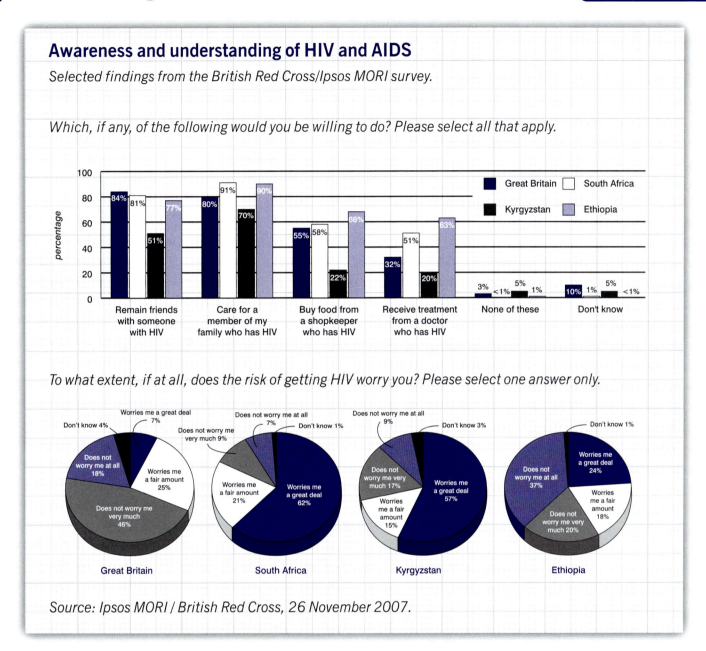

To what extent, if at all, does the risk of getting HIV worry you? Please select one answer only.

Source: Ipsos MORI / British Red Cross, 26 November 2007.

DID YOU KNOW?
Peer education programmes such as those run by the British Red Cross allow young people to learn about HIV and AIDS from other people their age, who have had special training to help them educate others about the disease.

Mini glossary

complacency – not being aware of danger

devastating – destructive, physically and emotionally

demystify – make clearer; make less mysterious

priority – most important task

promote – push forward; publicise

dignity – the state of having self-respect and the respect of others

www.redcross.org.uk/hiv

Living with HIV

ALISON WAS DIAGNOSED with the HIV virus when she was only 19.

My name's Alison and I am a 28-year-old heterosexual living near the south coast in England. I am pretty sure I became infected with HIV after a very unpleasant gap-year experience in Africa when I was 19.

On my return home, my GP arranged my HIV test and made sure that a local health advisor was available when I got my results, to give my mother and me support. This was all handled really sensitively, but was an incredibly stressful and traumatic experience in itself.

> I really fear discrimination and prejudice and this stops me from being open with most people and probably adds to the isolation I feel.

Since then my health has been fine and I am monitored by my local genito-urinary medicine (GUM) clinic a couple of times a year. I am lucky that I still haven't needed to go on to medication and I really hope this situation lasts as long as possible.

Personal feelings

I have told my closest friends and family and they have been great, but they don't really know what it is like to live with HIV. Over time I have managed to think about it less and less as this helps me not to worry and lets me get on with my life. But from time to time I get really scared about getting really ill – I guess I am a bit paranoid – and I do sink into a bit of a gloomy mood about it all.

Discrimination

I haven't experienced discrimination, but that is because I haven't been very open about my status. I really fear discrimination and prejudice and this stops me from being open with most people and probably adds to the isolation I feel. I feel stuck with my job as I know that they have an HIV non-disclosure and non-discrimination policy and a good pension. I don't know what I would face in another job.

Relationships

I only know one other person living with HIV, who is someone I met through the GUM clinic I was monitored at while I was at university. It made such a big difference meeting someone else who knew what I was going through.

The hardest thing was telling subsequent boyfriends. If you don't tell, you aren't having an honest relationship, so how can you really go anywhere with it? If you do tell and it's early days and doesn't work out, that is someone out there you can't really trust who knows something about you, which they could then use to ruin your life. It would make me feel so vulnerable.

I was so incredibly lucky to meet my now husband. I told him straight away. It was a gamble, but it meant that we were honest with each other from the start. He has been great and even got some information leaflets from THT to learn more about HIV. It makes me so sad that I will never be able to have unprotected sex with him.

Mini glossary

traumatic – mentally painful; difficult to deal with emotionally

monitored – regularly checked

paranoid – very afraid for no logical reason

isolation – state of being alone; loneliness

disclosure – revealing something

subsequent – following on; coming after

www.tht.org.uk

Activities

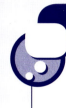

Brainstorm

Brainstorm to find out what you know about HIV and AIDS.

1. What is HIV?

    ....

    ....

2. What are the ways HIV can be passed from person to person?

    ....

    ....

3. What is the difference between HIV and AIDS?

    ....

    ....

Oral activities

4. 'If AIDS doesn't get them something else will' (see page 5). Discuss this in a group with relation to the AIDS crisis in developing countries. Does your group think it is a fair comment? Give your reasons.

    CONCLUSIONS...

    ....

    ....

5. 'This house believe that those who become infected with HIV through unprotected sex only have themselves to blame'. As a class, divide into two groups, with one group arguing in support of this motion and the other against.

    NOTES...

    ....

Moral Dilemmas

6. Read *The stigma of HIV and AIDS* on pages 10-11. How would you feel if a friend or family member told you they were HIV-positive? Would you be willing to remain friends with them? Give your reasons.

7. Since 2005, it has been illegal for employers to discriminate against people on the grounds that they are HIV-positive. Imagine you were an MP voting on this issue in Parliament. Do you agree that people living with HIV should be protected from discrimination in the same way as other disabled people? How would you have voted?

Activities

Research activities

8. Using the quiz on page 8 as a starting point, conduct interviews with people you know from a number of different groups, such as your friends, teachers and family members. What trends can you observe in the answers of people of different ages? Which age group is most well-informed about AIDS? Present your findings in a graph.

NOTES...

....

....

9. Using the Internet, do some research into the so-called 'Tainted Blood' scandal, in which thousands of haemophiliacs around the world were accidentally given HIV and Hepatitis C after being given transfusions of infected blood in the 70s and 80s. What were the major causes of this tragedy? Do you think something similar could ever happen again? How could it be prevented?

CONCLUSIONS ....

....

....

....

Written activities

Complete the following activities in your exercise books or on a sheet of paper.

10. Read *Living with HIV* on page 12. Write a poem from the 19-year-old Alison's point of view, exploring the emotions she might have felt on being told by the doctor that she was HIV positive. She describes the experience as 'stressful and traumatic' – would she feel angry, afraid, shocked?

11. Write a diary entry for a HIV-positive woman in a developing country who has just discovered she is pregnant. What would her hopes and fears for her unborn child be? Would she be aware of ART and how to access it? How well would she understand the HIV virus and how it is passed on?

Design activities

12. Create an informative leaflet which could be given to someone newly diagnosed as HIV-positive, covering any questions they may have about their condition. You may want to include information on changes they can expect to their health, antiretroviral HIV medicines and their legal rights in terms of employment and discrimination. You could also include information on life expectancy and progress towards finding a cure for AIDS, but remember to handle these issues sensitively.

Stop HIV: beyond ABC

Understanding HIV infection and prevention

HIV can only be passed on in a few ways: through sex, blood and mother-to-child transmission. Educating people about HIV and about the behaviours that put them at risk – such as unprotected sex and injection drug use – and helping them to behave safely are at the heart of HIV prevention. Yet, to stop HIV we need to understand what makes some people more vulnerable to HIV infection than others. Around the world, HIV is a disease of poverty and gender inequality. Statistics prove this: the highest rates of HIV occur in the poorest countries, where more women than men are infected, and young women are most at risk of getting HIV.

Lack of access to basic prevention services

According to UNAIDS, less than 20% of people at risk of HIV infection have access to basic prevention. Also, only 11% of the world's pregnant women have access to services to prevent mother-to-child transmission (PMTCT), even though this method of transmission is one of the cheapest and easiest to prevent. Providing more prevention services in 125 low- and middle-income countries would prevent over 28 million new HIV infections between now and 2015 – the target date for achieving the Millennium Development Goals.

Poverty and HIV/AIDS prevention

Because AIDS is a disease of poverty and because women are almost 70% of the world's poor, giving women more economic power can help HIV prevention. The main way this can be done is by making sure everyone has access to a free basic education. Primary education can reduce the effects of poverty, particularly on girls and women, decrease early marriage, encourage family planning, and increase equality between men and women and awareness of human rights – all of which can slow the spread of HIV.

Did you know?

With over 33 million people infected with HIV worldwide and over 7,400 new infections every day, access to HIV prevention services for everyone is essential. In 2007, about three million people became infected with HIV, including 470,000 children under the age of 15 (most infected through mother-to-child transmission of the virus). HIV prevention does not have to be complicated to make a big difference to the spread of HIV/AIDS. But it does have to address the different needs of all populations at risk – from injection drug users to adult married women.

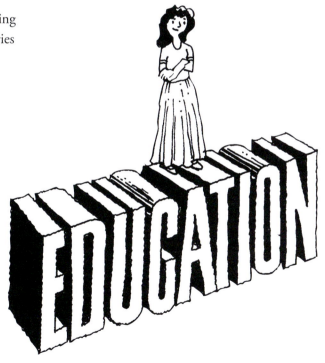

66 *To stop HIV we need to understand what makes some people more vulnerable to HIV infection than others.* **99**

Stop HIV: beyond ABC

Stopping sexual transmission of HIV

HIV prevention includes a wide range of programmes that have been scientifically proven. One common approach to HIV prevention is the 'ABC' model. ABC – **a**bstinence, **b**e faithful, use a **c**ondom – can be quite good at preventing the spread of HIV. However, for ABC to work, programmes that encourage abstinence and faithfulness must work together to delay the first time someone has sex and limit the number of sexual partners. At the same time, condom education programs teach teenagers and adults about safer sex and give them access to condoms. The reality is that most people become sexually active in their late teens, young girls in the global South are often forced into early marriages, and affairs outside of marriage are not uncommon. This means that everyone needs accurate information about how to protect themselves against HIV when they do have sex.

What needs to be done?

In order to meet the Millennium Development Goals by 2015, much more attention will need to be paid to the AIDS pandemic. As a result, United Nations member states have committed themselves to achieving specific targets for universal access to HIV/AIDS services by 2010. The targets include reducing AIDS cases by 25%, reducing the number of HIV-infected children by 50%, and increasing to 95% the percentage of young people who both correctly identify ways to prevent HIV and reject major myths about HIV. These commitments must be kept if we are to slow down and eventually reverse the spread of HIV/AIDS.

www.globalaidsalliance.org

The above information is reprinted with kind permission from the Global AIDS Alliance. © Global AIDS Alliance

Stopping intravenous transmission of HIV

Although unprotected sex remains the main way HIV is passed on worldwide, blood and injection safety is also a very important part of HIV prevention. Hundreds of thousands of HIV infections are caused each year through unsafe injections in healthcare settings; for example, through accidental needle pricks during vaccinations. Laboratory safety and access to clean syringes in health care settings are needed to prevent this method of HIV transmission. But encouraging safe behaviour among injection drug users (IDUs) is also important, and often overlooked. Nearly one-third of all HIV infections outside Africa are caused by injection drug use, yet only 5% of IDUs worldwide receive any HIV prevention services. Injection drug use is a very important factor in the HIV/AIDS epidemics of countries like Russia, China and Vietnam. Clean needle exchange and programmes to help people who wish to stop using injection drugs should be made widely available.

Prevention technologies

Finally, as HIV and AIDS continue to spread, destroying entire communities, it is very important that more is invested in new technologies to prevent HIV. Female condoms should be made available at low cost around the world. Research into microbicides, which would allow women to protect themselves against HIV without their partner's knowledge or cooperation, and into a vaccine for HIV should receive greater investment from the global community.

Mini glossary

gender inequality – a situation where men and women are not treated as equals by the society they live in

abstinence – stopping oneself from doing something which might be harmful: for example, not having sex

intravenous – into a vein

Treatment for HIV

THERE IS NO CURE FOR HIV. However, there are drugs that can stop HIV reproducing and can drive down the amount of the virus in the body to very low levels.

Combination therapy

Taking a combination of three or more drugs can stop HIV from reproducing and let the immune system recover. It also stops HIV changing its nature, or mutating, every time it reproduces.

Every copy of itself that HIV produces is a little bit different. HIV copies itself very fast, and quite often a copy of HIV will be produced that is not affected by one or more drugs. This is known as a resistant virus.

Side-effects

Many people experience short-term side-effects when they first start taking the drugs that they are prescribed, but these usually get better after a few weeks. Any long-term side-effects should be monitored by a doctor or clinic and dealt with if they occur.

Dangerous side-effects of anti-HIV drugs are rare, but if experienced a patient should see their doctor immediately.

Mini glossary

side-effects – effects of taking a medicine apart from its primary purpose

prescribed – when medicines are given which are only available by showing a document (prescription) signed by a doctor to a pharmacist

How combination therapy works

Different drugs stop HIV reproducing in different ways and a combination of three or more are needed to work. The aim of treatment is to reduce the amount of the virus to the lowest possible level, although it won't completely disappear.

There are now an increasing number of anti-HIV drugs for doctors to use in combination therapy.

www.tht.org.uk

The above information is reprinted with kind permission from the Terrence Higgins Trust. © Terrence Higgins Trust

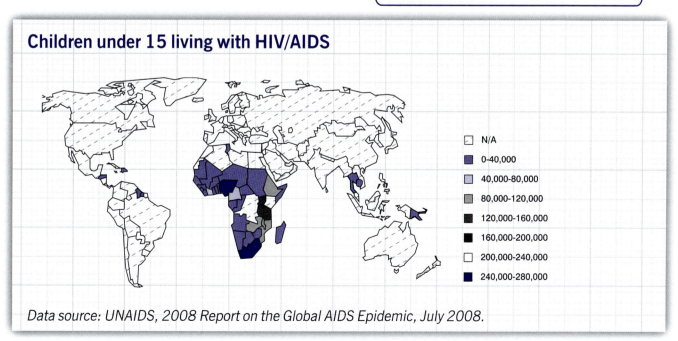

Children under 15 living with HIV/AIDS

Legend:
- N/A
- 0-40,000
- 40,000-80,000
- 80,000-120,000
- 120,000-160,000
- 160,000-200,000
- 200,000-240,000
- 240,000-280,000

Data source: UNAIDS, 2008 Report on the Global AIDS Epidemic, July 2008.

Protect the children

Did you know?

HIV/AIDS is having a big effect on children. Around the world, more than 15 million children under 18 have had one or both of their parents die from AIDS – a number that is expected to reach 20 million by 2010. In sub-Saharan Africa, 12 million children – 80% of the global total – have been made orphans by AIDS, and millions more live in households where an adult is sick.

Studies have found that orphans are more likely to be smaller than they should be and less likely to attend school than children living with both parents. A poor diet and little access to health services put orphans at higher risk of starvation, illness and death. And if they are not being looked after by a loving parent or guardian, the children may also be very unhappy.

> **" Around the world, more than 15 million children under 18 have had one or both of their parents die from AIDS – a number that is expected to reach 20 million by 2010. "**

Many AIDS orphans have HIV themselves, and around the world at least two million children under 15 are living with HIV/AIDS. Another 1,000 children are given HIV each day – most through mother-to-child transmission of the virus. Around the world, over 270,000 children die of AIDS each year, and in some countries the epidemic accounts for as many as half of all deaths among children under five.

Altogether, children under the age of 15 account for 14% of both AIDS-related deaths and new HIV infections worldwide. But only 6% of the approximately three million people now getting HIV treatment are children. And only 33% of HIV-positive pregnant women are getting antiretroviral medicine that can stop them passing the virus to their baby. Antiretroviral medicines made especially to treat children with AIDS can cost five times as much as adult versions, and are not as easy to get. Also, the expensive and complicated tests needed to find out if a child has HIV mean that half of HIV-infected

children die before their second birthday without anyone realising they had the infection.

HIV/AIDS is making the desperate situation of children worldwide worse. As the epidemic kills more and more adults, extended families are struggling to care for all the orphans. They have less money to spend on health, education, and healthy food. In households where adults have AIDS, older children often have to look after their families and care for the sick adult(s). Children of all ages struggle with the pain of losing a parent and the stigma of living in a family touched by HIV/AIDS. Even children who don't lose family members to AIDS may lose their teachers, doctors, neighbours, and other adult role models.

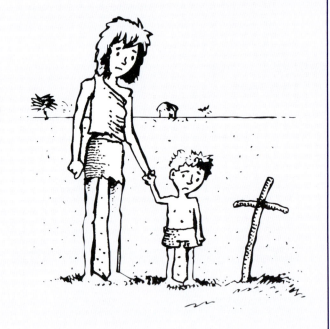

Although they are vulnerable, children have been forgotten about by organisations fighting HIV. According to UNICEF, less than 10% of children orphaned and made vulnerable by HIV/AIDS get any public support or services to help them. And just one in seven of the estimated 780,000 children who need antiretroviral therapy are getting treatment.

Protect the children

What needs to be done?

The most important first step in slowing down the AIDS epidemic among children is to prevent HIV being passed from pregnant mothers to their babies, and charities, companies and governments must do more to make prevention of mother-to-child transmission (PMTCT) programmes available where needed. Also, there needs to be more tests available for infants younger than 18 months, to find out if they have the HIV virus.

Orphans and vulnerable children (OVC), including children with HIV/AIDS, need care and support. This includes access to education, healthcare, housing, food and nutrition, and support within society. Orphans and vulnerable children also need special protection against abuse, violence and being badly treated in other ways. Giving medicine and care to parents with HIV/AIDS will help keep families together as long as possible, and, of course, children with HIV must be given treatment.

Also, families and local communities need help so they can raise orphans and vulnerable children in good homes.

Finally, all children must have access to a free, good basic education, and all children must be protected against violence that threatens their physical and emotional well-being and increases their risk of getting HIV.

> **The most important first step in slowing down the AIDS epidemic among children is to prevent HIV being passed from pregnant mothers to their babies.**

> **Around the world, more than 15 million children under 18 have had one or both of their parents die from AIDS.**

DID YOU KNOW? *Just one in seven of the estimated 780,000 children who need antiretroviral therapy are getting treatment.*

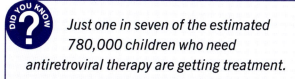

www.globalaidsalliance.org

Mini glossary

sub-Saharan Africa – *the area of the African continent which is to the south of the Sahara desert*

approximately – *not exact, but very close*

vulnerable – *unprotected; unable to take care of themselves*

estimated – *made an educated guess*

nutrition – *a balance of food in the amounts needed for good health*

Millions receiving HIV medicine

THREE MILLION PEOPLE are now receiving life-saving HIV drugs, but access to prevention and treatment is still lacking for millions.

The end of 2007 marks an important step in the history of the HIV/AIDS epidemic. Nearly three million people are now receiving antiretroviral therapy (ART) in low- and middle-income countries, a new report has said.

The report also shows other areas of progress, including improved access to services aimed at preventing mother-to-child transmission of HIV (PMTCT) and more testing and counselling.

Greater access: greater need

The authors state that about 31% of the estimated 9.7 million people in need of ART received it by the end of 2007. That means that an estimated 6.7 million in need are still unable to get these life-saving medicines.

Dr Peter Piot, Executive Director of UNAIDS, said:

66 This report highlights what can be achieved despite the many constraints that countries face and is a real step forward towards universal access to HIV prevention, treatment care and support. Building on this, countries and the international community must now also work together to strengthen both prevention and treatment efforts. 99

HIV-positive women who are able to access antiretroviral therapy while they are pregnant have a very low risk of passing on the infection to their baby during childbirth.

Millions now accessing treatment

According to the authors of the report, at the end of 2007 nearly 1 million more people (950,000) were receiving antiretroviral therapy – bringing the total number of people receiving ART to almost 3 million.

According to the report, the rapid increase of ART is due to a number of things, including the:

► increased availability of drugs, mostly because of price reductions;

► improved systems to get ART to the people who need it, tailored to the needs of individual countries;

► increased demand for ART as the number of people who are tested and diagnosed with HIV goes up.

Preventing HIV in children

At the end of 2007, nearly 500,000 women were able to access anti-retrovirals to stop them passing on HIV to their unborn children – up from 350,000 in 2006. During the same period, 200,000 children were receiving ART, compared to 127,000 at the end of 2006. The difficulty of diagnosing HIV in infants, however, is a big obstacle in the way of further progress.

66 *The authors state that about 31% of the estimated 9.7 million people in need of ART received it by the end of 2007. That means that an estimated 6.7 million in need are still unable to get these life-saving medicines.* 99

Millions receiving HIV medicine

UNICEF Executive Director Ann M. Veneman said:

❝ We are seeing encouraging progress in the prevention of HIV transmission from mother to newborn. The report should motivate us to focus and redouble our efforts on behalf of children and families affected by HIV/AIDS. ❞

DID YOU KNOW?

Tuberculosis, or TB, is a highly infectious disease which usually affects the lungs. It is spread through the air when people cough or sneeze, and can be fatal. It is now very rare in the UK but is still common in some other countries. One in four deaths from TB is HIV-related.

Mini glossary

constraints – *limitations; things which restrict freedom*

universal – *available to everyone*

motivate – *give a reason to take action*

tuberculosis (TB) – *an infectious disease, often fatal*

integrated – *combined; brought together*

www.who.int

The above information is reprinted with kind permission from the World Health Organisation. © World Health Organisation

Tuberculosis and weak healthcare systems slow progress

Other obstacles to providing more treatment include patients leaving many treatment programmes when treatment is still needed and the large numbers of individuals who do not know that they have HIV, or are diagnosed too late and die in the first six months of treatment.

Tuberculosis is a leading cause of death among HIV-infected people worldwide, and the number one cause of death among those living in Africa. Healthcare services dealing with tuberculosis are often not integrated with those dealing with HIV. Too many people are losing their lives because they are unable to either prevent TB or access life-saving medications for both TB and HIV.

❝ *Tuberculosis is a leading cause of death among HIV-infected people worldwide.* ❞

The authors of the report warn that widening access to ART is likely to be slow due to weak health systems in the worst-affected countries, especially the difficulty of training and keeping healthcare workers. Healthcare systems in regions where the AIDS epidemic is worse become weaker because of 'brain drain', where skilled healthcare workers move to other occupations and countries. Healthcare workers are also lost due to high mortality rates from HIV itself.

2 June 2008

HIV patients living longer

PEOPLE WITH HIV IN WEALTHY COUNTRIES are living about 13 years longer due to improvements in combination antiretroviral therapy (cART), according to new research by the University of Bristol.

Improvements in cART mean life expectancy has gone up by about 13 years from 1996-99 to 2003-05. However, life expectancy in HIV-positive people is still much lower than the population in general, and HIV patients who do not start treatment until later have worse life expectancy.

Since cART was introduced in 1996, the way it is given to patients has been continually improved. However, the effect of HIV on life expectancy since combination therapy has been available is not very well understood. This is because the treatment is still so new.

Academics from Bristol University and other institutions compared changes in mortality and life expectancy among HIV-positive individuals taking cART.

Patients treated later after becoming infected had shorter life expectancy, at 32.4 years, compared with 50.4 years in patients treated at earlier stages.*

Patients who probably got HIV by injecting drugs had a shorter life expectancy (32.6 years) than those from other groups (44.7 years). Finally, women had a slightly longer life expectancy than men (44.2 v 42.8 years), probably because women on average start their HIV treatment earlier after becoming infected.*

Although the results are encouraging, an HIV-positive person starting cART at age 20 will only, on average, live another 43 years (to age 63), while a 20-year-old HIV-negative person in a wealthy country can expect to live to around 80 years, a difference of nearly 20 years. The study authors have asked for improved health services and living conditions for HIV patients to help close the gap.

* The figures given in these paragraphs refer to the further life expectancy of someone aged 20. So for example, a person with a life expectancy of 32.6 years at age 20 is expected to live until they are 52.6 years old overall.

Professor Sterne, one of the study authors, said:

❝ The progressive reductions in mortality and gains in life expectancy over the three periods studied here are probably the result of both improvements in therapy during the first decade of cART and continuing declines in mortality rates among individuals on such treatment for long periods. These advances have transformed HIV from being a fatal disease, which was the reality for patients before the advent of combination treatment, into a long-term chronic condition.

The results of this study indicate that people living with HIV in high-income countries can expect increasing positive health outcomes on cART. The marked increase in life expectancy since 1996 is a testament to the gradual improvement and overall success of such treatment. ❞

25 July 2008

www.bristol.ac.uk

Mini glossary

life expectancy – *the amount of time someone can expect to live*

mortality – *frequency of death; rate at which death occurs in a certain section of the population*

progressive – *making progress*

chronic – *lasting a long time*

testament – *something which can be used as proof or evidence of a fact*

A cure for AIDS

THERE IS NO CURE FOR AIDS. Although antiretroviral medicines can hold back HIV – the virus that causes AIDS – and can delay illness for many years, it cannot kill the virus completely. There is no confirmed case of a person getting rid of HIV infection. Sadly, this doesn't stop countless quacks and con artists selling unproven, often dangerous 'AIDS cures' to desperate people.

It is easy to see why an HIV-positive person might want to believe in an AIDS cure. It is hard to get antiretroviral treatment in much of the world. When someone has a life-threatening illness they may want to believe in anything they think will help them stay alive. And even when antiretroviral treatment is available, it is not an easy solution. Drugs must be taken every day for the rest of a person's life, often causing unpleasant side effects. A one-off cure to get rid of the virus once and for all is much more attractive.

Distrust of Western medicine is not uncommon, especially in developing countries. The Internet is full of rumours of the pharmaceutical industry or the US government concealing AIDS cures to protect the market for patented drugs. Many people would prefer a remedy that is 'natural' or 'traditional'.

Where's the harm in fake AIDS cures?

Unproven AIDS cures have been around since the disease was discovered in the early 1980s. In most cases, they have only made suffering worse.

First of all, fake cures are a swindle. Someone who invests their savings in a worthless potion or an electrical zapper has less money to spend on real medicines and healthy food.

Many sellers of fake cures insist their clients avoid all other treatments, including antiretroviral medicines. By the time a patient realises the 'cure' hasn't worked, it may be too late for them to start antiretroviral treatment which could extend their life.

Fake cures may also cause direct harm to health. Inventors often refuse to reveal their recipes. Some so-called cures have been found to contain industrial chemicals, disinfectants and other poisons.

Finally, the promotion of fake AIDS cures undermines HIV prevention. People who believe in a cure are less likely to fear becoming infected with HIV, and therefore less likely to behave safely.

> **Distrust of Western medicine is not uncommon, especially in developing countries.**

ARV treatment worldwide

What is the regional breakdown of people receiving antiretroviral (ARV) treatment?

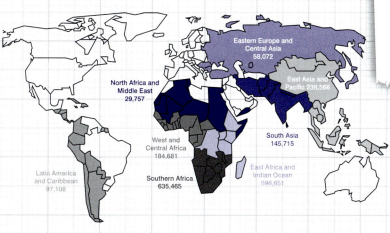

Eastern Europe and Central Asia
58,072

North Africa and Middle East
29,757

East Asia and Pacific 238,566

West and Central Africa
184,681

South Asia
145,715

Latin America and Caribbean
97,108

Southern Africa
635,465

East Africa and Indian Ocean
596,651

Source: Global Fund ARV Fact Sheet, 1 December 2008. The Global Fund to Fight AIDS, Tuberculosis and Malaria

A cure for AIDS

Respected research on curing AIDS

A wide range of actions – including such extreme measures as bone marrow transplantation – have failed in trials to kill off HIV infection. Currently, many researchers believe the best way would be to combine antiretroviral treatment with drugs that flush HIV from its hiding places. The idea is to force resting CD4 cells to become active, when they will start producing new HIV particles. The activated cells should soon die or be destroyed by the immune system, and the antiretroviral medication should mop up the released HIV.

Early attempts to do this used interleukin-2 (also known as IL-2 or by the brand name Proleukin). This chemical messenger tells the body to create more CD4 cells and to activate resting cells. Researchers who gave interleukin-2 together with antiretroviral treatment discovered they could no longer find any infected resting CD4 cells. But interleukin-2 failed to clear all of the HIV; as soon as the patients stopped taking antiretroviral drugs the virus came back again.

❝ There is a lot about HIV that remains unknown. ❞

There is a problem with creating a large number of active CD4 cells: despite the antiretroviral drugs, HIV may manage to infect a few of these cells and replicate, keeping the infection alive. Scientists are now investigating chemicals that don't activate all resting CD4 cells, but only the few that are infected with HIV.

One such chemical is valproic acid, a drug already used to treat epilepsy and other conditions. In 2005, a group of researchers led by David Margolis caused a sensation when they reported that valproic acid, combined with antiretroviral treatment, had greatly reduced the number

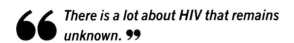

Some so-called AIDS 'cures' have been found to contain industrial chemicals, disinfectants and other harmful poisons.

Why is it so difficult to cure AIDS?

Curing AIDS is usually taken to mean clearing the body of HIV, the virus that causes AIDS. The virus replicates (makes new copies of itself) by inserting its genetic code into human cells, particularly a type known as CD4 cells. Usually the infected cells produce lots of HIV particles and die soon afterwards. Antiretroviral drugs interfere with this replication process, which is why the drugs are so good at reducing the amount of HIV in a person's body to very low levels. During treatment, the amount of HIV in the blood often falls so low that it cannot be detected by the standard test, known as a viral load test.

Unfortunately, not all infected cells behave the same way. Probably the most important problem is caused by 'resting' CD4 cells. Once infected with HIV, these cells, instead of producing new copies of the virus, lie inactive for many years. Current therapies cannot remove HIV's genetic material from these cells. Even if someone takes antiretroviral drugs for many years they will still have some HIV hiding in parts of their body. Studies have found that if treatment is removed then HIV can re-establish itself by leaking out of these 'viral reservoirs'.

A cure for AIDS must somehow remove every single one of the infected cells.

of HIV-infected resting CD4 cells in three of four patients. They concluded that:

'This finding, though not definitive, suggests that new approaches will allow the cure of HIV in the future.'

Sadly, more recent studies have suggested that valproic acid has no long-term benefits. In fact it's quite possible that no treatment based on 'flushing out' the virus from resting CD4 cells will work because the virus has other hiding places besides these cells. There is a lot about HIV that remains unknown.

A cure for AIDS

Some of the world's top research institutions are now trying to learn more about the behaviour of HIV, resting CD4 cells and other hiding places. But the truth is that HIV research does not receive a lot of funding. Some people think the search for a cure is not worth much investment because it could be impossible to find one.

❝ *Unproven AIDS cures have been around since the disease was discovered in the early 1980s. In most cases, they have only made suffering worse.* ❞

Yet there are still those who remain hopeful, including the research charity amfAR, which in 2006 gave nearly $1.5 million to AIDS cure researchers.

Activist Martin Delaney is among those calling for an end to negative attitudes:

❝ Far too many people with HIV, as well as their doctors, have accepted the notion that a cure is not likely. No one can be certain that a cure will be found. No one can predict the future. But one thing is certain: if we allow pessimism about a cure to dominate our thinking, we surely won't get one… We must restore our belief in a cure and make it one of the central demands of our activism. ❞

The above information is reprinted with kind permission from AVERT. © AVERT

www.avert.org

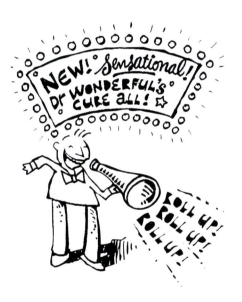

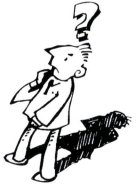

Mini glossary

quacks – people pretending to be medical doctors and giving false health advice

con artists – criminals who use tricks to gain someone's confidence, usually in order to get money from them

pharmaceutical industry – the industry which produces medicines and disease treatments

patented – something which is only allowed to be produced and sold by one person or company

swindle – a trick which cons someone out of their money

undermines – weakens or damages

definitive – 100% reliable; giving a final solution

pessimism – a tendency to predict the worse

Activities

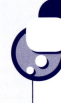

Brainstorm

Brainstorm to find out what you know about tackling the AIDS problem.

1. How can the spread of AIDS be stopped?

    ....

    ....

2. What treatments are there for HIV-positive people?

    ....

    ....

Oral activities

3. What do you think are some of the reasons people in developing countries continue to have unprotected sex when AIDS causes so many deaths? Compare your list with a partner's and discuss how the issues you have highlighted could be addressed to tackle the AIDS epidemic.

    ....

    ....

    ....

4. Read *A cure for AIDS* on pages 23-25. Why is the promotion of fake AIDS cures dangerous? Role play a situation in which a doctor tries to explain gently to an HIV-positive person in the developing world that there is no cure for their condition and discourages them from buying fake cures.

    NOTES...

    ....

Moral Dilemmas

5. 'People with HIV are going to die anyway so there is no point investing money in medicine for them. Instead, the money should be spent on finding a cure for the disease.' Do you agree or disagree with this statement? Give your reasons.

6. The head of the Catholic Church, Pope Benedict, has sparked debate by refusing to endorse condom use in Africa. Catholics do not agree with using condoms because they believe the purpose of sex is to reproduce, but HIV is mainly spread through unprotected sex. A fifth of Africans are Catholic, and 22 million Africans are HIV positive. How do you feel about this issue? Is the Pope right or wrong?

Activities

Research activities

7. Find out more about the work of the Global AIDS Alliance (start by visiting their website: www. globalaidsalliance.org). What do they think are the main problems which need addressing in the fight against AIDS? How are they working to fight the epidemic? How effective have their efforts been so far?

CONCLUSIONS ....

....

....

....

8. Use the Internet to find out more about the Millennium Development Goals. What are they and how will they help fight AIDS? Are they likely to be met? Use your research as the basis for an article for your school magazine titled 'AIDS and the Millennium Development Goals'.

NOTES ....

....

....

....

Written activities

Complete the following activities in your exercise books or on a sheet of paper.

9. Read *Protect the children* on pages 18-19. Summarise the problem of HIV and AIDS for children in the developing world in less than 350 words.

10. Read *Stop HIV: beyond ABC* on pages 15-17. Which groups of people are most at risk of getting HIV worldwide? Do charities seeking to tackle the AIDS crisis need to target their prevention efforts differently to different groups? Draw up and fill in a table with columns titled 'At risk group', 'Reasons for increased risk' and 'Best prevention strategy'.

Design activities

11. Imagine you are producing a leaflet which will be used by British Red Cross peer educators to help explain the HIV virus to children and young people in developing countries. Design your leaflet, including some simple information on what HIV and AIDS are, how to prevent them being spread and how antiretroviral medicines work. You may like to include simple diagrams showing how HIV infects CD4 white blood cells and how ART medicines slow down the progress of the infection.

Key Facts

▶ Worldwide, it is estimated that over 40 million people are living with HIV and around three million people die each year from AIDS-related illnesses. (page 1)

▶ HIV infection can be passed through blood, semen, breast milk and vaginal fluids. HIV can't be passed on through normal day-to-day activities, such as sharing cutlery, sitting on toilet seats or by shaking hands. (page 1)

▶ The HIV virus weakens the immune system so that eventually it can no longer fight diseases – this is called having AIDS. People with AIDS can die of illnesses which the immune system might normally be able to fight off, such as pneumonia. (page 2)

▶ The latest statistics from the Health Protection Agency show that the number of people living with HIV in the UK went up to an estimated 77,400 in 2007, with 7,734 new diagnoses in 2007 alone. (page 6)

▶ Over a quarter (28 per cent) of people living with HIV don't know they have the infection and many of those that are diagnosed are being diagnosed late – after the point at which they should have started treatment. (page 7)

▶ Research published on 26 November 2007 shows that one in seven young people interviewed in Britain would not be willing to stay friends with someone if they had HIV and only 32% are worried about getting HIV. (page 10)

▶ According to UNAIDS, less than 20% of people at risk of HIV infection have access to basic prevention. Only 11% of the world's pregnant women have access to services to prevent mother-to-child transmission (PMTCT). (page 15)

▶ There is no cure for HIV. However, there are drugs that can stop HIV reproducing and can drive down the amount of the virus in the body to very low levels. (page 17)

▶ Around the world, more than 15 million children under 18 have had one or both of their parents die from AIDS – a number that is expected to reach 20 million by 2010. (page 18)

▶ Just one in seven of the estimated 780,000 children who need antiretroviral therapy are getting treatment. (page 19)

▶ The authors of a new report have stated that about 31% of the estimated 9.7 million people in need of ART received it by the end of 2007. That means that an estimated 6.7 million in need are still unable to get these life-saving medicines. (page 20)

▶ People with HIV in wealthy countries are living about 13 years longer due to improvements in combination antiretroviral therapy (cART), according to new research by the University of Bristol. (page 22)

Glossary

The ABC strategy – This was a sex education policy designed to combat the HIV and AIDS epidemic in Africa – Abstinence, Be faithful, use a Condom.

AIDS – Acquired Immune Deficiency Syndrome. AIDS is diagnosed when the immune system has been weakened so much by HIV that it cannot fight certain life threatening infections and illnesses. It is fatal and cannot be cured.

Anti-retroviral therapy (ART) – Treatment for the HIV virus which can slow down the progress of the illness and delay it from becoming AIDS. Those who have access to ART treatment can live a lot longer than those who don't, but many people with HIV in developing countries are often not able to get the medicine.

Epidemic – When there are a lot more cases of a disease than might be expected in a certain area, it is called an epidemic. Epidemics can be very difficult to control, with the disease quickly spreading to more and more people. AIDS is said to be an epidemic in some parts of the world.

HIV – Human Immunodeficiency Virus. An infection that can be passed from person to person through unprotected sex, from needles contaminated with infected blood, through blood transfusion or organ donation from people with the virus and from mother to baby. HIV affects the body's immune system, weakening its ability to fight infection.

Immune system – The immune system protects your body against infection. A key part is white blood cells. These cells find and destroy invading germs, such as bacteria and viruses, preventing serious diseases and damage to your body. HIV avoids being destroyed by the immune system by repeatedly changing its outer 'coat'. It multiplies (replicates) within the special type of white blood cells called CD4 cells. These cells are normally involved in helping other types of immune cell to attack and destroy disease-causing germs. As HIV multiplies, it destroys CD4 cells, so there are less of them. The reduction in CD4 cells means that the body's ability to fight infection is weakened.

Millennium Development Goals – A set of aims set out in 2000 when world leaders decided that they needed a strategy to tackle poverty. They set and agreed targets, which are called the Millennium Development Goals. Goal 6 aims to have halted and begun to reverse the spread of HIV/AIDS by 2015.

Pandemic – Like an epidemic, except a pandemic is not confined to a certain region: a disease pandemic can spread very quickly across large areas such as continents.

Stigma – When someone is treated badly or has judgements made about them because they have a certain characteristic which other people do not approve of. There is a stigma surrounding HIV, and many of those who have the disease are treated badly because other people are not well-educated about HIV and think they will catch it by sharing water glasses or shaking hands. Some people may also think HIV patients have lots of sexual partners, use drugs or are gay, even though they may not belong to any of these higher-risk groups.

Transmission – Passing something from one person to another.

Vaccine – Medicine which, once given, means a person will never catch a certain disease.